POST-MENOPAUSE SEX GUIDE

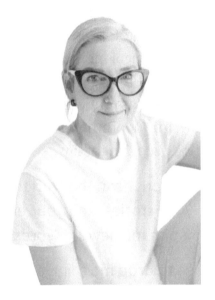

How to Stay Intimate and Satisfied

COPYRIGHT © 2023

[Amara Adams]

Dear readers, you mean the world to me. Your feedback, your stories, and your experiences inspire me beyond words.

Feel free to drop me a line anytime at insightfuladam007@gmail.com. I would be absolutely delighted to hear from you!

TABLE OF CONTENT

INTRODUCTION

Embracing Post-Menopausal Intimacy

Navigating the waters of post-menopausal intimacy can be both exciting and challenging. As we move beyond a significant phase in life, the dynamics of our relationships and sense of undergoing self transformation shifts. It's at this juncture that we must confront the vital topic of intimacy with renewed vigor and understanding.

Intimacy: A Journey Beyond Menopause

Consider representing the diverse facets of our lives as a lush garden in bloom. Just as seasons change, so do our experiences— menopause marking a significant transition. The concept of intimacy takes on new dimensions, intertwining with personal growth and emotional fulfillment. This guide aims to be your compass, guiding you through uncharted territories and helping you embrace the beauty of intimacy post-menopause.

A Conversation Worth Having

Imagine sitting across a dear friend, sipping tea on a cozy porch. The conversation turns intimate as you share stories, laughter, and insights. Similarly, this book seeks to foster a comfortable, open dialogue about the shifts in intimacy that come with menopause. It's an exploration, a journey, and a conversation—both with yourself and your partner.

The Power of Embracing Change

Change is the essence of life itself, and menopause is an integral part of that change. Through our shared experiences, we'll uncover the power that lies in embracing these changes. By acknowledging and understanding the transformations within ourselves, we pave the way for enriching, vibrant relationships.

Why This Guide Matters

In a world where discussions about intimacy can still carry stigma, it's time to shatter the silence. As a self-improvement advocate and someone deeply invested in offering practical solutions, I've embarked on this journey to help you navigate post-menopausal intimacy. Together, we'll unravel the complexities, dispel myths, and celebrate the beauty of connection that transcends age.

Join me in this exploration of post-menopausal intimacy—a journey of rediscovery, connection, and profound growth. Let's begin by diving into the heart of what it means to stay intimate and satisfied beyond menopause.

Thought-Provoking Questions - Reflecting on Intimacy and Transformation

As we embark on this transformative journey through post-menopausal intimacy, let's delve into a series of thought-provoking questions that invite you to ponder, explore, and uncover the layers of your own experiences:

1. What does intimacy mean to you in the context of your current life stage?

2. How have societal perceptions about aging impacted your view of post-menopausal intimacy?

3. Can you recall a moment when you felt a deep, emotional connection with a partner or loved one? How has that connection evolved over time?

4. In what ways has your relationship with yourself changed as you've transitioned through menopause?

5. Imagine embracing intimacy as an evolving journey rather than a destination. How does this shift in perspective resonate with you?

6. Have you experienced any apprehensions or anxieties about addressing intimacy after menopause? What strategies have you used to navigate these feelings?

7. Consider a time when you've felt truly comfortable discussing intimate topics. What factors contributed to that comfort, and how can you recreate that environment for deeper conversations?

8. How do you envision post-menopausal intimacy enhancing other aspects of your life, such as your sense of self, emotional well-being, and overall relationship dynamics?

9. If you could describe the essence of post-menopausal intimacy using just three words, what would they be?

10. Imagine looking back on this phase of life a decade from now. What advice would you give to your present self about embracing intimacy with grace and enthusiasm?

These thought-provoking questions serve as gateways to introspection, guiding you to explore the corners of your thoughts and feelings about post-menopausal intimacy. Through reflection, we can uncover insights that shape our understanding, enhance our connections, and inspire positive change. As we continue this journey, keep these questions in mind, allowing them to spark meaningful conversations with yourself and those around you.

Personal Anecdote - My Journey to Unveiling Post-Menopausal Intimacy

Embarking on the path to writing "The Post-Menopause Sex Guide: How to Stay Intimate and Satisfied" was a journey that mirrored the transformative nature of the topic itself. Here's a glimpse into the inspiration behind this guide:

Picture a tranquil morning, sunlight filtering through a canopy of trees as I sit down to write. It was during one of these moments that the idea for this guide first took root. As a passionate advocate for personal growth and meaningful connections, I found myself drawn to the often uncharted territory of post-menopausal intimacy. The curiosity was driven by a desire to address a topic that, despite its significance, often remains veiled in silence.

Reflecting on my own experiences and conversations with readers, I realized that the landscape of intimacy changes after menopause—just as our lives do. The concept of intimacy expands beyond the physical, intertwining with emotional growth, communication, and the art of embracing change. This guide was born out of a determination to fill the gap in resources that speak directly to this journey, offering guidance that's empathetic, empowering, and deeply personal.

Throughout my research and interactions, I encountered stories of resilience, transformation, and rekindled connections that underscored the importance of this guide. It's not just about addressing physical changes; it's about embracing the essence of what makes us human—our desire for connection, growth, and understanding.

As I navigated the process of crafting this guide, I found myself enriched by the stories and experiences of individuals who graciously shared their insights. Their journeys became intertwined with mine, and this book became a collective effort—an exploration of the human experience that celebrates the power of vulnerability and transformation.

Now, as you embark on the pages of this guide, I invite you to join me on a journey of discovery, empowerment, and profound growth. Let's dive into the heart of post-menopausal intimacy together, armed with personal insights, practical solutions, and the understanding that intimacy is a journey to be embraced at every stage of life.

Overview of the Book's Purpose and Structure - Guiding You Through the Landscape of Post-Menopausal Intimacy

In "The Post-Menopause Sex Guide: How to Stay Intimate and Satisfied," our journey is more than just a collection of words on pages; it's a pathway to empowerment, understanding, and joyful connection. This book is designed to be your trusted companion as you navigate the intricate realm of post-menopausal intimacy, offering insights, guidance, and practical solutions that resonate with your personal growth journey.

Purpose of the Book: Navigating Intimacy Beyond Menopause

This guide is a response to a profound need—the need for a comprehensive resource that addresses the multifaceted dimensions of intimacy after menopause. Its purpose is to empower you to embrace the changes that come with this life stage and to inspire a positive outlook on the transformative power of intimacy. Through personal insights, thought-provoking questions, and actionable advice, the book aims to help you foster deeper connections, both with yourself and your partner.

Structure of the Book: Mapping Your Journey

Chapter 1: Embracing Change Dive into the heart of menopause's impact on intimacy. Explore societal perceptions, common myths, and the beauty of embracing change. Discover how embracing transformation sets the stage for a fulfilling journey.

Chapter 2: Navigating Communication Communication is the cornerstone of any thriving relationship. This chapter equips you with tools to foster open, meaningful conversations about intimacy with your partner, guided by real-life stories and empathetic insights.

Chapter 3: Rediscovering Desire Delve into the concept of desire as it evolves through menopause. Drawing on personal anecdotes and relatable metaphors, this chapter helps you reconnect with your desires, nurturing a deeper sense of self.

Chapter 4: Physical Well-being and Pleasure Leverage your expertise in health and fitness as we explore the intertwining of physical well-being and pleasure post-menopause. Through practical exercises and actionable advice, discover ways to enhance your physical comfort and enjoyment.

Chapter 5: Emotional Intimacy Uncover the significance of emotional intimacy and its profound impact on relationships. With personal stories and engaging exercises, learn to foster deeper emotional connections that transcend age and circumstance.

Chapter 6: Overcoming Obstacles Challenges are an inherent part of any journey. This chapter addresses potential obstacles and offers practical strategies, punctuated by success stories, that empower you to overcome hurdles with grace.

Chapter 7: Celebrating Connection As the journey unfolds, reflect on the transformation and growth you've experienced. Summarize key takeaways, celebrate your progress, and apply the wisdom gained from the pages of this guide.

Your Empowering Path Forward Conclude with a heartfelt message, reminding you of your capacity to navigate post-menopausal intimacy with confidence. This section encourages ongoing growth, exploration, and a deep connection with your own journey.

As we embark on this journey together, I invite you to immerse yourself in the pages of this guide, to reflect, engage, and embrace the powerful connection that intimacy offers in the post-menopausal phase of life. This book is designed to be your roadmap—a guide that marries practicality with personal insights, resonating with your aspirations for growth, connection, and satisfaction.

CHAPTER 1

Embracing Change - Navigating the Transformations of Menopause

Menopause's Impact on Intimacy: Understanding the Journey Ahead

Menopause, a natural and inevitable phase of a woman's life, ushers in a period of change that extends beyond its physical implications. This chapter is dedicated to exploring the intricate tapestry of both physical and emotional transformations that accompany menopause, and how they intersect with the realm of intimacy.

The Physical Transition

Menopause signifies the culmination of the reproductive years, marked by the cessation of menstruation. This biological transition is orchestrated by hormonal changes, particularly the decrease in estrogen and progesterone levels. These hormonal shifts give rise to a range of physical changes that can impact both physical comfort and sexual experiences.

- Vaginal Changes: Reduced estrogen levels can lead to vaginal dryness, thinning of vaginal walls, and changes in pH levels. These factors may contribute to discomfort during intercourse and affect overall sexual well-being.

- Sexual Response: Hormonal fluctuations can influence sexual desire, arousal, and even orgasm. Understanding these shifts is key to navigating changes in sexual experiences.

- Physical Comfort: Hot flashes, night sweats, and sleep disturbances are common during menopause, potentially affecting overall energy levels and quality of life.

The Emotional Landscape

Menopause's impact extends beyond the physical realm, intertwining with emotional well-being and self-perception.

- Emotional Fluctuations: Hormonal changes can lead to mood swings, anxiety, and even depression. It's crucial to recognize that these emotional fluctuations are a natural part of the journey.

- Self-Image: Menopause can sometimes evoke feelings of loss or diminished self-esteem due to societal perceptions. Realigning self-perception and embracing this new phase are essential steps towards maintaining healthy relationships.

- Partner Dynamics: Both partners may experience adjustments as menopause unfolds. Effective communication and mutual understanding become pivotal in navigating this period together.

Why Embrace Change?

The journey through menopause is more than a series of challenges; it's an opportunity for growth, exploration, and deeper connections. Embracing these changes is about fostering a renewed sense of self, strengthening relationships, and redefining intimacy in ways that celebrate this new chapter.

As we progress through this chapter, we'll navigate the landscape of post-menopausal intimacy with empathy, curiosity, and a commitment to understanding the holistic transformations that shape this phase of life. By acknowledging the interplay between physical and emotional changes, we empower ourselves to not just endure, but to thrive during this journey of embracing change.

Dispelling Misconceptions - Redefining Intimacy Beyond Menopause

Navigating the landscape of post-menopausal intimacy requires confronting the misconceptions and societal perceptions that often cloud our understanding. By addressing these myths head-on, we can pave the way for a more empowered, fulfilling journey:

Myth 1: Intimacy Fades Away

One of the most common misconceptions is that intimacy dwindles after menopause. The truth is, intimacy is a dynamic force that evolves, taking on new forms that are just as meaningful and fulfilling. While physical aspects might shift, emotional connections can flourish, fostering a deeper bond between partners.

Myth 2: Desire Disappears

A prevailing belief is that desire disappears with menopause. In reality, desire transforms and adapts. It might manifest in less predictable ways, driven more by emotional connection and shared experiences. By embracing this evolution, we open ourselves to discovering new dimensions of intimacy.

Myth 3: Aging Diminishes Appeal

Society often perpetuates the notion that aging diminishes attractiveness, affecting self-esteem and inhibiting intimate connections. The truth is, attractiveness transcends age. Confidence, self-assuredness, and the wisdom acquired over time can exude an allure that deepens connections and fosters intimacy.

Myth 4: Physical Changes Hinder Pleasure

The physical changes that come with menopause can lead to the misconception that pleasure is compromised. However, with open communication, adaptability, and a willingness to explore, pleasure can be redefined and experienced in new, fulfilling ways. Intimacy becomes an opportunity for creative and shared growth.

Myth 5: Intimacy Becomes Irrelevant

Society sometimes reinforces the idea that post-menopausal intimacy becomes irrelevant in the face of other life priorities. Yet, intimacy remains a crucial component of holistic well-being. It contributes to emotional health, self-expression, and the sense of connection that enhances overall life satisfaction.

Redefining the Narrative

It's time to rewrite the narrative surrounding post-menopausal intimacy. By shedding light on these misconceptions, we empower ourselves to embrace change with authenticity and enthusiasm. This chapter serves as a platform for unraveling these unhelpful beliefs, recognizing that intimacy is a journey that transcends age and is enriched by experience.

In the pages ahead, we'll continue to explore the transformations that menopause brings and how they intersect with intimacy. By dismantling these myths and redefining perceptions, we create space for growth, learning, and the genuine connections that thrive when grounded in truth. Let's journey forward with a clear understanding, fostering intimacy that is as vibrant and meaningful as the lives we lead.

Personal Insight - Navigating Intimacy: A Personal Story

Allow me to share a personal experience that underscores the power of navigating intimacy during the post-menopausal phase. My hope is that this story resonates with you, offering insights and reassurance as you embark on your own journey of rediscovery:

The Garden of Transformation

In the midst of my own exploration of post-menopausal intimacy, I found myself drawn to a garden that became a metaphor for this transformative phase. Just as a garden experiences seasons of change, our lives also ebb and flow through various stages. I reflected on the beauty that emerges from embracing each season, even as the landscape transforms.

During a visit to this garden, I encountered a magnificent tree that had stood the test of time. Its branches, once heavy with vibrant blooms, had shed their petals, giving way to a more intricate pattern of branches and leaves. I was reminded that growth isn't always outward; sometimes it's in the delicate intricacies that unfold within.

As I stood there, observing the tree's resilience, I realized that the tree's journey mirrored our own. **Menopause isn't a departure from intimacy—it's a shift towards a different kind of intimacy.** Just as the tree's transformation fostered new forms of life, our evolution during this phase can deepen connections and create new paths of emotional intimacy.

The Power of Connection

In conversations with women navigating this journey, I encountered a story that beautifully captured the essence of post-menopausal intimacy. A couple shared their experience of redefining connection. They spoke of open conversations, mutual understanding, and an appreciation for the evolving nature of desire. Their journey wasn't about clinging to the past, but about embracing the present with a renewed sense of curiosity and exploration.

Their story illustrated that the power of intimacy lies not solely in the physical, but in the emotional bonds we forge. It's about the laughter shared, the vulnerabilities exchanged, and the growth experienced together. Their journey was a testament to the fact that change can lead to connection—a connection that deepens as they navigate the intricacies of life's different seasons.

Your Journey Ahead

As you navigate the chapters of this guide, I encourage you to view your journey through the lens of this personal story. Embrace the shifts, both physical and emotional, as opportunities for growth and connection. Just as the garden flourishes through change, so can your intimate relationships. With each chapter, we'll dive deeper into the strategies, insights, and personal anecdotes that illuminate the path ahead.

Remember, this journey is uniquely yours, shaped by your experiences, desires, and aspirations. By embarking on this voyage with an open heart and a willingness to embrace change, you're fostering the foundations of lasting and meaningful intimacy. As we continue forward, keep in mind the tree, the garden, and the transformative power of embracing each season with authenticity and grace.

Navigating the changes that menopause brings to intimacy requires a blend of insight and practicality. Here, we'll explore actionable tips that can guide you on your journey of acceptance and empowerment:

1. Open Communication: The foundation of any successful relationship is communication. Initiate open and honest conversations with your partner about the changes you're experiencing. Sharing your thoughts, concerns, and desires can lead to a deeper understanding and mutual support.

2. Educate Yourself: Knowledge is empowering. Spend some time learning about the mental and emotional changes that come with menopause. Understanding the science behind these shifts can help dispel myths and reduce anxiety.

3. Prioritize Self-Care: Self-care is an essential component of embracing change. Engage in activities that nourish your physical and emotional well-being, whether it's practicing mindfulness, engaging in regular exercise, or exploring new hobbies.

4. Embrace Pleasure: Embrace the exploration of pleasure in all its forms. This includes understanding your body's changing needs and discovering what brings you joy and satisfaction. It's about fostering a positive relationship with your body and celebrating the journey it's on.

5. Experiment and Adapt: Be open to trying new things. Experiment with different forms of intimacy, communication styles, and activities that foster connection. Adaptability is key, as you discover what works best for you and your partner.

6. Seek Professional Support: If you find that challenges persist, consider seeking the guidance of a healthcare professional or therapist specializing in sexual health. Their expertise can provide personalized solutions and support tailored to your unique needs.

7. Embrace Emotional Intimacy: Remember that intimacy extends beyond the physical. Emotional intimacy, built on trust, vulnerability, and mutual understanding, can foster deeper connections that transcend the physical changes.

8. Set Realistic Expectations: Embrace change with realistic expectations. Understand that the journey might involve ups and downs, and that both you and your partner are adapting. Approach each experience with an open mind.

9. Practice Self-Compassion: Be kind to yourself. Menopause is a transformative phase that involves both challenges and growth. Embrace self-compassion as you navigate the path of change, recognizing that you're on a journey of discovery.

10. Celebrate Progress: Celebrate your progress, both big and small. Recognize the steps you've taken to embrace change, deepen connections, and foster growth. Each effort contributes to a more empowered and fulfilling journey.

Remember, embracing change isn't about erasing the past—it's about integrating new experiences into the rich tapestry of your life. By combining practical strategies with an open heart, you're forging a path towards intimacy that's grounded in understanding, empathy, and a shared commitment to growth. As we continue to explore the chapters ahead, keep these tips in mind, knowing that you have the tools to navigate this transformative journey with grace and empowerment.

CHAPTER 2

The Power of Open Communication

Communication serves as the heartbeat of any healthy relationship. When it comes to post-menopausal intimacy, open dialogue becomes even more essential. In this section, we'll delve into the significance of fostering honest and empathetic conversations with your partner about the changes that accompany this phase:

The Unspoken Divide

Imagine a bridge connecting two sides of a beautiful landscape. Effective communication serves as that bridge, linking partners emotionally, mentally, and intimately. However, the landscape of post-menopausal intimacy can be marked by unspoken concerns, societal taboos, and misconceptions. This unspoken divide has the potential to weaken connections and hinder growth.

Breaking the Silence

Open communication is the antidote to this divide. It creates an environment where both partners can openly share their thoughts, desires, and concerns without fear of judgment. By initiating these conversations, you're fostering a sense of safety that encourages vulnerability and mutual understanding.

The Significance of Vulnerability

Vulnerability is often viewed as a sign of strength rather than weakness. Sharing your thoughts and feelings about post-menopausal intimacy requires vulnerability, allowing you and your partner to deepen your emotional connection. It's through vulnerability that true growth and meaningful change can take root.

Setting the Stage for Conversations

Creating a Safe Space

Begin by creating a safe environment for dialogue. Find a comfortable and private setting where you can engage in an uninterrupted conversation. Setting the stage in this way fosters an atmosphere of trust and encourages candid sharing.

Choosing the Right Time

Timing matters. Choose a moment when both you and your partner are relaxed and receptive. Avoid discussing intimate matters in high-stress situations or when time is limited. Prioritize creating an atmosphere conducive to genuine conversation.

Active Listening

Communication is a two-way street. Actively listen to your partner's thoughts and concerns without interruption or judgment. Reflecting back what you've heard and asking follow-up questions demonstrates your engagement and willingness to understand.

Using "I" Statements

Frame your thoughts using "I" statements to express your feelings and experiences without sounding accusatory. For example, say "I feel" instead of "You always." This approach promotes personal responsibility for your feelings and encourages a non-confrontational dialogue.

Navigating Sensitive Conversations

Starting the Conversation

Initiating the conversation might feel daunting, but remember that you're both on this journey together. You might begin by expressing your desire for openness and growth in your relationship. Sharing your intent sets a positive tone for the conversation.

Discussing Desires and Concerns

Approach the conversation by sharing your desires and concerns, both emotional and physical. Be candid about what you're experiencing and the changes you're navigating. Encourage your partner to share their thoughts as well, creating a platform for mutual understanding.

Handling Challenges

Challenges might arise during these conversations. Your partner's response might differ from your expectations, but remember that open communication is a process. Be patient, and practice active listening and empathy even in the face of differing viewpoints.

Building a Shared Vision

As you navigate post-menopausal intimacy, work together to build a shared vision of what your intimate relationship can look like. This vision will serve as a guidepost as you explore new avenues of connection and growth.

Cultivating Connection

Ultimately, the significance of open communication is about cultivating a deeper connection. It's about fostering a partnership where both partners feel heard, valued, and supported. As you embark on these conversations, remember that you're creating a foundation for a more intimate, empathetic, and resilient relationship—one that embraces change with open arms.

By embracing open communication, you're not only addressing the challenges of post-menopausal intimacy but also nurturing a bond that grows stronger through shared vulnerability and understanding. In the chapters ahead, we'll delve further into strategies for nurturing this connection and exploring new dimensions of post-menopausal intimacy together.

Real-Life Stories of Successful Communication

Stories that Illuminate the Power of Dialogue

Real-life stories serve as beacons of inspiration, reminding us of the transformative power of open communication. Here are two stories that shine a light on how couples navigated post-menopausal intimacy through dialogue:

The Journey of Shared Discovery

Meet Sarah and James—an inseparable couple who had spent decades building a life together. As menopause approached, Sarah noticed shifts in her desires and physical comfort. Instead of letting these changes drive a wedge between them, Sarah decided to initiate a conversation.

One evening, after sharing a quiet dinner at home, Sarah gently broached the topic. She expressed her feelings openly, sharing her hopes for continued closeness and her uncertainties about the changes. James, eager to support Sarah, listened attentively. Together, they embarked on a journey of shared discovery.

Through open communication, Sarah and James learned to embrace the changes as opportunities for exploration. They researched, experimented, and found new ways to kindle their connection. James became an enthusiastic partner in understanding Sarah's evolving desires, and their intimacy flourished in ways they never anticipated.

Redefining Connection Through Compassion

Lucy and Mark, a couple who had weathered life's challenges together, found themselves at a crossroads as Lucy entered menopause. Lucy's changing body triggered self-doubt and discomfort, which she initially kept to herself. However, her emotional struggles began to affect their intimacy.

One day, Mark gently approached Lucy with his concerns, expressing his desire to support her. Lucy, touched by his compassion, opened up about her feelings of vulnerability. Mark reassured Lucy of his unwavering love and commitment and expressed his eagerness to learn and adapt alongside her.

Their conversation marked a turning point. Lucy and Mark embarked on a joint effort to understand and address Lucy's concerns. Mark's empathetic approach created a safe space for Lucy to express her thoughts, fears, and desires. With his support, Lucy felt empowered to explore solutions, ultimately finding renewed confidence in their connection.

The Lessons We Can Learn

These real-life stories underscore the transformative potential of open communication. They remind us that successful conversations are grounded in empathy, mutual support, and a shared commitment to growth. Here are some key takeaways from these stories:

Listening is Empathy: Both partners in each story actively listened and empathized with one another. This laid the foundation for understanding and partnership.

Vulnerability Fuels Growth: Sharing vulnerabilities paves the way for growth and connection. Vulnerability breeds authenticity and encourages partners to adapt and explore together.

Partnership in Change: In both stories, couples embarked on a shared journey of discovery. By recognizing that they were in this together, they forged a path of mutual exploration and adaptation.

Adaptability is Key: Successful communication involves adapting to changes together. A willingness to learn and grow enhances emotional intimacy and strengthens the bond between partners.

As you reflect on these stories, remember that every couple's journey is unique. Embrace the lessons they offer and apply them in ways that resonate with your relationship. By fostering open communication, you're fostering the growth of a bond that can weather life's changes with grace and resilience. In the chapters ahead, we'll continue to explore strategies for deepening connections and navigating post-menopausal intimacy together.

Navigating Sensitive Conversations - Starters and Techniques

Initiating Conversations with Sensitivity

Navigating sensitive conversations requires a delicate touch and thoughtful approach. Here, we'll explore conversation starters and techniques designed to foster understanding and encourage open dialogue about post-menopausal intimacy:

Conversation Starter 1: "I've been reflecting on our journey together, and I believe our intimacy deserves an open conversation. Can we discuss how we can navigate this phase of life while deepening our connection?"

This opener sets a positive tone, emphasizing your desire for growth and partnership. It invites your partner to engage in the conversation with empathy and curiosity.

Conversation Starter 2: "I value our connection and want us to continue thriving together. Let's explore how we can adapt to the changes we're experiencing and uncover new avenues of intimacy."

By framing the conversation in terms of shared growth, you're highlighting your commitment to a mutually fulfilling relationship. This approach encourages collaboration and mutual support.

Techniques for Open and Constructive Dialogue

Technique 1: Active Listening

Active listening is a cornerstone of effective communication. Give your partner your full attention, make eye contact, and avoid interrupting. Show that you're engaged by nodding and using verbal cues like "I understand" or "Tell me more."

Technique 2: Reflective Responses

Responding reflectively demonstrates that you're truly engaged in the conversation. Repeat back what your partner has said in your own words to ensure you've understood correctly. For instance, "If I'm hearing you correctly, you're feeling uncertain about the changes we're going through?"

Technique 3: Using "I" Statements

Use "I" statements to express your feelings and thoughts without assigning blame. For instance, "I've noticed changes in my body that I'm still adapting to. I wanted to talk about how we can navigate this journey together."

Technique 4: Ask Open-Ended Questions

Open-ended questions encourage deeper exploration. Instead of asking yes-or-no questions, pose inquiries that invite your partner to share their thoughts and feelings. For example, "How do you envision our intimate connection evolving during this phase?"

Technique 5: Validate Emotions

Validation is key to making your partner feel heard and understood. Acknowledge their feelings and emotions, even if they differ from your own. For instance, "It sounds like you're feeling a mix of uncertainty and curiosity about this phase, which is completely valid."

Technique 6: Plan Regular Check-Ins

Set aside time for regular check-ins dedicated to discussing intimate matters. These scheduled conversations create a safe space for ongoing dialogue, preventing concerns from being pushed aside.

Navigating Discomfort

Technique 7: Dealing with Discomfort

Sensitive conversations can sometimes trigger discomfort. Acknowledge the discomfort, but don't let it deter you from engaging. Recognize that growth often emerges from stepping outside your comfort zone.

Technique 8: Give Each Other Grace

Approach sensitive conversations with patience and understanding. Recognize that both you and your partner are navigating uncharted territory. Give each other grace to express feelings and adapt at your own pace.

By utilizing these conversation starters and techniques, you're fostering an environment where intimate dialogue can thrive. Navigating sensitive topics requires empathy, active listening, and a commitment to growth. As we continue through this chapter, keep these tools in mind, knowing that you have the resources to embark on conversations that deepen your connection and empower your post-menopausal intimacy journey.

Creating a Safe and Supportive Space for Dialogue

Nurturing a Safe Haven for Intimate Conversations

The significance of open communication is magnified when it takes place within a safe and supportive environment. In this section, we'll delve into the importance of creating such a space for intimate dialogue about post-menopausal intimacy:

A Sanctuary of Trust

Imagine a sanctuary—a place where vulnerability is met with empathy, where concerns are greeted with understanding, and where growth is nurtured. Creating a safe space for dialogue is akin to building this sanctuary within your relationship—a haven where both partners can share openly without fear of judgment.

Embracing Vulnerability

Vulnerability is the cornerstone of intimacy. When you establish a safe space, you're inviting your partner to share their thoughts, feelings, and uncertainties without hesitation. This environment encourages authenticity, paving the way for deeper connections and mutual growth.

Why Safety Matters

A safe space sets the stage for transformative conversations. It:

Fosters Trust: Trust is cultivated when partners feel heard and supported. A safe environment reinforces the understanding that both partners are on the same team, navigating challenges together.

Reduces Fear of Judgment: The fear of judgment can hinder open communication. When partners feel safe, this fear is diminished, allowing for candid conversations without apprehension.

Encourages Empathy: A safe space encourages active listening and empathy. Partners are more likely to consider each other's feelings and viewpoints, enriching the quality of the conversation.

Guidelines for Creating a Safe Space

Creating a safe space involves intentional efforts to establish trust and empathy:

Mutual Respect: Approach conversations with respect for each other's feelings and experiences. Value your partner's perspective as much as your own.

Non-Judgmental Attitude: Refrain from passing judgment or assigning blame. Focus on understanding and finding solutions together.

Active Listening: Give your partner your full attention when they talk. Listen not only to respond, but to also understand.

Express Empathy: Validate your partner's feelings by expressing empathy. Let them know you understand their perspective, even if you don't share the same feelings.

Time and Patience: Allow time for conversations to unfold naturally. Avoid rushing or forcing discussions before both partners are ready.

Setting Boundaries: Respect each other's boundaries regarding when and how conversations take place. Ensure both partners feel comfortable.

Embracing the Journey Together

Creating a safe and supportive space for dialogue about post-menopausal intimacy is an ongoing endeavor. It requires commitment, empathy, and a shared understanding of its significance. Remember that this space is a haven—a place where growth, exploration, and understanding flourish.

As we navigate the chapters ahead, keep the concept of this sanctuary in mind. By fostering an environment of safety and support, you're embarking on a transformative journey—one that has the potential to reshape your relationship and post-menopausal intimacy in profound and beautiful ways.

CHAPTER 3

Rediscovering Desire - Navigating Intimacy's New Horizon

The Evolution of Desire in the Menopausal Journey

Desire, a complex and multifaceted aspect of intimacy, undergoes a unique transformation during the menopausal journey. In this section, we'll delve into the concept of desire, exploring how it evolves and takes on new dimensions during this transformative phase:

Understanding Desire

Desire, often defined as a yearning or longing for connection and intimacy, is a cornerstone of human relationships. It's the spark that ignites passionate connections, the magnetic force that draws partners together, and the foundation upon which physical and emotional intimacy is built.

The Menopausal Shift

As menopause ushers in its physical and emotional changes, desire undergoes a shift that calls for a fresh perspective. Hormonal fluctuations can lead to changes in desire, arousal, and even sexual response. While these changes might initially seem unfamiliar, they're part of a natural evolution—a transition that invites partners to explore desire in new and meaningful ways.

Embracing the Ebb and Flow

Desire's transformation during menopause often involves an ebb and flow—an ebbing of traditional patterns and a flowing towards uncharted territories. This fluidity invites couples to reframe their understanding of desire and to navigate this journey together with curiosity and empathy.

Navigating Desire's New Landscape

Discovering Emotional Intimacy

Menopause calls for a shift from the physicality of desire to the realm of emotional intimacy. While traditional markers of desire might evolve, the longing for connection remains constant. Emotional intimacy—fostered through communication, vulnerability, and shared experiences—takes center stage.

Cultivating Desire through Connection

The journey of rediscovering desire involves cultivating it through connection. Partners are invited to explore new ways of fostering closeness, whether through shared hobbies, deep conversations, or acts of affection. These interactions serve as fertile ground for desire to flourish.

Honoring Personal Needs

Individual needs within a relationship play a crucial role in the evolution of desire. Partners are encouraged to communicate their personal desires, explore their unique interests, and create a space where their individual passions can contribute to the shared experience of intimacy.

Finding Beauty in Change

Embracing the transformation of desire is about finding beauty in change. It's recognizing that desire isn't a static entity, but a living force that evolves with us. By honoring this evolution, couples open themselves to the potential for growth, exploration, and a deeper connection that transcends physicality.

A New Chapter of Exploration

The evolution of desire during menopause signifies a new chapter of exploration—an invitation to redefine what intimacy means. This journey requires partners to embrace vulnerability, communicate openly, and approach desire with a sense of curiosity and adventure.

As we journey through this chapter, remember that desire's transformation isn't a departure from intimacy, but an opportunity to reinvent and revitalize it. By navigating this new landscape with empathy and open hearts, you're embarking on a voyage of rediscovery—one that has the potential to deepen your connection and create a more profound sense of intimacy than ever before.

Metaphors of Desire's Evolution

Navigating Desire's New Landscape Through Metaphors

Metaphors offer us a unique lens through which we can view complex concepts. Let's explore the evolution of desire during menopause through relatable metaphors that paint a vivid picture of this transformative journey:

Metaphor 1: The Shifting Tides of a River

Imagine desire as a river that has journeyed through various terrains. During menopause, this river encounters a change in landscape. The currents might ebb and flow differently, carving new pathways. Just as the river doesn't lose its essence, desire remains an essential part of the journey. It takes on a different rhythm, flowing through uncharted territories, and creating new spaces of intimacy.

Metaphor 2: The Seasons of a Garden

Consider desire as a garden that experiences different seasons. Menopause brings a shift from the vibrant bloom of spring to the reflective tranquility of autumn. The garden doesn't lose its beauty—it transforms, offering a unique palette of colors and textures. Similarly, desire doesn't vanish; it evolves into a different expression, fostering emotional connections and moments of shared growth.

Metaphor 3: The Pages of a Book

Envision desire as a book with chapters that evolve over time. Menopause introduces a new chapter—a departure from the familiar plotlines. The narrative might be less about intensity and more about depth. Just as a book's essence remains intact, desire's core endures. It becomes a story of exploration, with pages that invite partners to delve into unexplored emotions and create new meaning in their intimacy.

Metaphor 4: The Symphony of Music

Think of desire as a symphony that shifts its melody. Menopause introduces new notes, creating a composition that resonates with emotional chords. The symphony doesn't lose its harmony—it evolves, weaving a tapestry of emotional connection. Just as the music captures our hearts in different ways, the evolution of desire captures partners' emotions in new and poignant dimensions.

Metaphor 5: The Constellations in the Sky

Imagine desire as constellations in the night sky. Menopause changes the arrangement, creating new patterns of connection. The constellations don't disappear; they become part of a new cosmic arrangement. Similarly, desire remains a guiding light— albeit in a different form. Partners navigate this celestial journey together, exploring the stars of emotional intimacy.

Lessons from Metaphors

These metaphors illuminate the evolution of desire during menopause, emphasizing continuity amidst transformation. They offer valuable lessons:

Change Isn't Loss: Just as nature evolves, so does desire. The metaphors remind us that change doesn't erase what was; it adds depth and new dimensions to our experiences.

Embrace the New: Metaphors highlight the beauty of embracing the new landscape. Desire's transformation invites partners to discover uncharted realms of connection.

Connection Remains: Like the river's essence, the garden's beauty, the book's story, the symphony's harmony, and the constellations' glow, the essence of desire remains. It takes on new forms, fostering emotional intimacy.

Celebrate Growth: Just as metaphors capture transitions, partners can celebrate the growth that comes with embracing the evolution of desire. It's an opportunity for partners to adapt, learn, and deepen their bond.

As you reflect on these metaphors, remember that they mirror the nuanced journey of desire's transformation. By embracing these metaphors, you're opening the door to a more profound and resilient intimacy—one that transcends the physical and embraces the emotional landscape of this transformative phase.

Personal Insights on Rediscovering Desire and Fulfilling Intimacy

Navigating Intimacy from a Personal Perspective

Navigating the landscape of rediscovering desire and maintaining a fulfilling sex life during menopause involves not only insights from experts but also personal experiences that shed light on this transformative journey. Here, I'll share personal insights drawn from my own journey of exploration:

Rediscovering Desire as a Journey

As I navigated the path of menopause, I came to realize that desire isn't a static destination—it's a journey of constant discovery. Rather than searching for what once was, I embraced the idea of finding new facets of desire that resonated with the woman I was becoming.

The Power of Emotional Intimacy

While physical desire underwent changes, the beauty of emotional intimacy emerged as a cornerstone of connection. Conversations that delved into dreams, shared memories, and even vulnerabilities became gateways to a deeper and more fulfilling intimacy.

Exploring New Pathways of Pleasure

As traditional markers of physical desire evolved, I found joy in exploring new pathways of pleasure. I let curiosity guide me, allowing myself to experiment with activities that sparked joy and connection, fostering a sense of adventure within my partnership.

Prioritizing Communication

Open dialogue became a lifeline during this journey. My partner and I recognized that communication wasn't just about addressing concerns—it was about celebrating victories and sharing desires. The more we communicated, the more we discovered our evolving desires and learned to embrace the changes together.

Adapting with Patience

Menopause taught me the value of patience. Adapting to changes wasn't instantaneous; it required patience and mutual support. We celebrated small victories and gave ourselves permission to explore at our own pace, allowing growth to unfold organically.

Championing Self-Care

I discovered the importance of self-care as a foundation for intimacy. Nurturing my physical and emotional well-being became an act of self-love that flowed into my intimate connection with my partner. Prioritizing self-care became an expression of the love I had for both myself and my relationship.

Embracing the New Normal

Above all, my journey of rediscovering desire led me to embrace the "new normal" with an open heart. Rather than clinging to past expectations, I chose to welcome change as an opportunity for evolution. This perspective allowed us to forge a path of intimacy that was uniquely ours.

Section 4: The Beauty of Personal Insight

These personal insights offer a window into the experience of navigating desire and intimacy during menopause. They underscore the value of embracing change, nurturing emotional connection, and fostering an environment of mutual support and growth. As you explore this chapter, keep these insights in mind, knowing that your personal journey of rediscovery holds the potential for a more profound and fulfilling intimacy—one that evolves with authenticity, love, and a sense of adventure.

Exercises for Reconnecting with Your Desires

Nurturing Intimacy Through Exploration

Rediscovering desire during menopause involves embarking on a journey of self-discovery and connection. Here, we'll explore exercises and activities designed to help you reconnect with your desires, fostering a deeper sense of intimacy and self-awareness:

Exercise 1: Reflecting on Desires

Take a quiet moment to reflect on your desires. Journal about what once ignited your passion and what you're curious about exploring now. Consider both physical and emotional desires, allowing your thoughts to flow freely.

Exercise 2: Dreaming Together

Engage in a shared activity where you both dream about the future. It could be a cozy evening at home or a leisurely walk outdoors. Discuss your hopes and desires for the years ahead, creating a space for open conversation and shared aspirations.

Exercise 3: Sensory Exploration

Reconnect with your senses through a sensory exploration exercise. Blindfold one another and take turns guiding each other through touch, taste, smell, and sound experiences. This exercise fosters a heightened sense of presence and connection.

Exercise 4: Memory Lane

Spend an evening reminiscing about your shared history. Go through old photographs, letters, or mementos that capture moments of joy, connection, and desire. Reflect on how these memories have shaped your journey together.

Exercise 5: Intimate Wishlist

Create an intimate wishlist together. Each partner writes down activities, experiences, or desires they'd like to explore. Share your lists and find common ground, creating a roadmap for cultivating new forms of intimacy.

Exercise 6: Sensual Exploration

Engage in a sensual exploration activity that encourages connection without pressure. This could involve a gentle massage, exploring new textures, or experimenting with different scents. The focus is on creating shared moments of relaxation and connection.

Exercise 7: Sharing Fantasies

Set aside time to share your fantasies with one another. Create a safe space where you can openly express your desires, creating a sense of vulnerability and intimacy. This exercise encourages partners to explore new dimensions of their connection.

Exercise 8: Love Letter Exchange

Write heartfelt love letters to each other, expressing your desires, feelings, and dreams. Exchange the letters in a private moment, creating an intimate connection through words that celebrate your journey together.

Exercise 9: Date Night with a Twist

Infuse your date night with an element of surprise. Plan an activity or experience that you wouldn't typically consider. This exercise encourages you to step outside your comfort zones and fosters a sense of shared adventure.

Exercise 10: Mindful Connection

Engage in a mindfulness exercise together, such as deep breathing or guided meditation. This practice creates a calm and centered atmosphere, allowing you to reconnect with your desires from a place of presence.

Embrace the Journey of Reconnection

These exercises offer a canvas upon which you and your partner can paint the colors of desire, connection, and exploration. Approach them with an open heart and a spirit of curiosity, knowing that each activity has the potential to reignite the spark of intimacy and create a deeper bond during this transformative phase. As you journey through this chapter, remember that the road to reconnection is uniquely yours to explore and embrace.

CHAPTER 4

Physical Well-being and Pleasure - Nurturing Your Body Through Change

Embracing Physical Well-being in the Menopausal Journey

As menopause introduces changes to your body, prioritizing physical well-being becomes an essential aspect of maintaining a fulfilling and vibrant life. In this section, we'll explore actionable advice and strategies for nurturing your body through this transformative phase:

1. Mindful Movement

Engage in regular physical activity that brings joy and energy to your body. Explore activities such as yoga, walking, swimming, or dancing. Focus on movement that nurtures both your physical and emotional well-being, helping you stay active and connected to your body.

2. Nutrient-Rich Eating

Opt for a balanced and nutrient-rich diet that supports your body's changing needs. Incorporate whole foods, lean proteins, fruits, vegetables, and healthy fats into your meals. Prioritize foods rich in calcium and vitamin D to support bone health, and consider incorporating phytoestrogen-rich foods like flaxseeds and soy.

3. Hydration and Self-Care

Stay hydrated by drinking plenty of water throughout the day. Hydration supports overall well-being, including skin health and digestion. Additionally, integrate self-care practices into your routine, such as enjoying a relaxing bath, practicing deep breathing, or engaging in mindfulness meditation.

4. Strength Training

Incorporate strength training exercises into your fitness routine. Building and maintaining muscle mass is important for bone health, metabolism, and overall strength. Consult a fitness professional to create a tailored strength training plan that suits your needs and goals.

5. Pelvic Floor Health

Prioritize pelvic floor health through exercises that strengthen these muscles. Pelvic floor exercises can support bladder control, enhance intimacy, and contribute to overall well-being. Consult a healthcare professional or pelvic floor specialist for guidance on exercises that are right for you.

6. Sleep Hygiene

Prioritize quality sleep by practicing good sleep hygiene. Create a comfortable sleep environment, establish a regular sleep schedule, and avoid stimulants before bedtime. Adequate sleep supports hormonal balance, mood regulation, and overall vitality.

7. Regular Health Check-ups

Schedule regular health check-ups with your healthcare provider. Regular screenings and consultations can help you monitor your overall health, address any concerns, and make informed decisions about your well-being.

8. Stress Management

Practice stress management techniques to support your physical health. Engage in activities that help you relax, such as meditation, deep breathing, or spending time in nature. Managing stress positively impacts hormonal balance and overall vitality.

9. Intimacy and Pleasure

Prioritize intimacy and pleasure as integral components of physical well-being. Engage in open communication with your partner, explore new avenues of connection, and embrace activities that foster emotional and physical intimacy.

10. Self-Compassion

Above all, practice self-compassion as you navigate this phase of change. Listen to your body, honor its needs, and celebrate its resilience. Embrace physical well-being as a journey of self-love and empowerment.

Navigating Physical Transformation

The journey of physical well-being during menopause involves embracing change, nurturing your body, and celebrating its strength. As we move through this chapter, remember that each step you take towards prioritizing your physical health is a step towards creating a more vibrant and fulfilling life post-menopause.

Navigating Physical Transformation - Expert Insights

Cultivating Physical Well-being Through Expert Perspectives

As a self-publishing author and blogger passionate about health, fitness, and well-being, I draw upon my expertise to offer relevant insights into navigating the physical transformation that accompanies menopause. Here, I provide expert advice and strategies to support your journey of nurturing your body during this transformative phase:

1. Hormonal Balance and Nutrition

During menopause, hormonal changes can impact your metabolism and body composition. Prioritize balanced nutrition with a focus on nutrient-dense foods. Incorporate lean proteins, fiber-rich carbohydrates, and healthy fats into your meals. Phytoestrogen-rich foods like soy, flaxseeds, and legumes can help support hormonal balance.

2. Bone Health and Exercise

Maintaining strong bones is crucial during menopause, as hormonal changes can lead to decreased bone density. Engage in weight-bearing exercises like walking, jogging, or weight lifting to promote bone health. Ensure you're getting adequate calcium and vitamin D through your diet or supplements.

3. Cardiovascular Health

Estrogen plays a protective role in cardiovascular health, and its decline during menopause can impact heart health. Engage in cardiovascular exercises like brisk walking, swimming, or cycling to support heart health. Prioritize whole foods that promote heart health, such as berries, fatty fish, nuts, and whole grains.

4. Strength Training and Muscle Mass

Loss of muscle mass is a common concern during menopause. Incorporate strength training exercises into your routine to preserve and build lean muscle. Resistance exercises using weights, resistance bands, or body weight can help improve muscle strength and metabolism.

5. Mind-Body Connection

Embrace mind-body practices like yoga, meditation, and deep breathing to manage stress and promote overall well-being. These practices can have a positive impact on hormonal balance and emotional health, contributing to a smoother menopausal transition.

6. Hydration and Skin Health

Stay hydrated to support skin health and overall well-being. Hydration plays a role in skin elasticity and can help alleviate common menopausal symptoms like dry skin. Consuming water-rich foods like fruits and vegetables can contribute to hydration.

7. Sleep Quality

Prioritize quality sleep, as sleep disturbances are common during menopause. Establish a bedtime routine, create a comfortable sleep environment, and limit screen time before bed. Adequate sleep supports hormonal balance, mood regulation, and overall vitality.

8. Intimacy and Emotional Well-being

Physical well-being is closely intertwined with emotional health and intimacy. Open communication with your partner and exploring activities that foster emotional connection can positively impact both physical and emotional well-being.

9. Professional Guidance

Consider seeking guidance from healthcare professionals, nutritionists, or fitness experts who specialize in menopause-related health. Individualized advice can help you tailor your wellness journey to your unique needs and goals.

10. Celebrate Your Strength

As you navigate physical changes, celebrate your body's strength and resilience. Embrace each step you take towards nurturing your well-being as an empowering act of self-care and self-love.

Embarking on Your Wellness Journey

Combining expert insights with your dedication to well-being sets the stage for a transformative journey. The strategies and advice provided in this section empower you to embrace physical well-being as an opportunity for growth, vitality, and connection during the menopausal transition. As you continue through this chapter, remember that you possess the knowledge and determination to nurture your body with care and intention.

Enhancing Pleasure and Comfort - Practical Techniques

Elevating Intimate Experiences Through Practical Methods

Enhancing pleasure and comfort during menopause involves exploring practical techniques that prioritize your well-being and intimacy. Here, I offer actionable exercises and strategies to enrich your intimate experiences and promote comfort during this transformative phase:

1. Sensate Focus Technique

Engage in the sensate focus technique, a mindfulness-based exercise that focuses on sensory awareness. With your partner, take turns exploring each other's bodies through touch. This exercise fosters a deeper connection and intimacy by focusing on sensation rather than performance.

2. Lubrication and Moisturizers

Use water-based lubricants and vaginal moisturizers to enhance comfort and pleasure. These products can alleviate dryness and discomfort, making intimate experiences more enjoyable. Choose products that are free from irritants and compatible with your body.

3. Communication and Consent

Prioritize open communication and mutual consent with your partner. Discuss desires, boundaries, and preferences before engaging in intimate activities. This establishes a foundation of trust and ensures both partners feel comfortable and respected.

4. Experimentation and Exploration

Embrace a spirit of experimentation and exploration. Try new activities, positions, or forms of touch that cater to your comfort and pleasure. This curiosity-driven approach can lead to delightful discoveries that enhance your intimate connection.

5. Relaxation Techniques

Incorporate relaxation techniques before engaging in intimate activities. Deep breathing, progressive muscle relaxation, or guided imagery can help reduce tension and create a calm and comfortable environment.

6. Pelvic Floor Exercises

Engage in pelvic floor exercises to strengthen the muscles that support bladder and vaginal health. These exercises, often referred to as Kegels, can enhance sensation and contribute to overall comfort during intimate experiences.

7. Warm Baths or Compresses

Enjoy warm baths or use warm compresses to relax pelvic muscles and promote blood flow to the genital area. This can alleviate tension and discomfort, creating a more relaxed and pleasurable experience.

8. Mindful Touch and Connection

Practice mindful touch by focusing on the present moment during intimate interactions. Tune into the sensations you're experiencing and the connection you're sharing with your partner. This mindfulness can enhance pleasure and emotional intimacy.

9. Set the Mood

Create a comfortable and inviting atmosphere for intimacy. Dim lighting, soft music, and comfortable bedding can contribute to a relaxing and pleasurable environment.

10. Educate Yourself

Educate yourself about the changes your body undergoes during menopause. Understanding the physical and emotional aspects of this phase can help you approach intimacy with knowledge and confidence.

Nurturing Intimate Bonds

By incorporating these practical techniques into your intimate experiences, you're fostering a connection that prioritizes pleasure, comfort, and emotional intimacy. As you journey through this chapter, remember that your willingness to explore, communicate, and nurture your intimate bond has the potential to create a more fulfilling and pleasurable post-menopausal journey.

Personal Experiences of Prioritizing Pleasure and Physical Activity

Navigating Pleasure and Movement Through Personal Insights

As someone deeply passionate about health, fitness, and well-being, I want to share my personal experiences related to staying physically active and prioritizing pleasure during menopause. These insights are drawn from my journey of exploration and self-discovery, and I hope they resonate with you as you embark on your own path:

1. Embracing Movement with Joy

Staying physically active during menopause has been a transformative journey for me. I discovered that movement isn't just about exercise; it's an expression of self-care and joy. Whether it's a brisk walk in the morning or a dance session in the living room, each moment of movement becomes an opportunity to celebrate my body's strength and vitality.

2. Connecting with Nature

One of the most rewarding aspects of staying active has been my connection with nature. Taking hikes, biking through scenic trails, or practicing yoga outdoors has allowed me to experience the rejuvenating power of nature. It's a reminder that movement isn't confined to a gym; it's a way to connect with the world around us.

3. Rediscovering Pleasure in Movement

Prioritizing pleasure in movement has been a game-changer. I learned to choose activities that bring me joy, whether it's dancing, swimming, or practicing tai chi. By focusing on activities that light up my spirit, I've created a sustainable and fulfilling fitness routine that supports my physical and emotional well-being.

4. Intimate Connection Through Movement

Movement has also deepened my connection with my partner. Engaging in activities like partner yoga or going for walks together has allowed us to share moments of connection and intimacy. Exploring movement as a team has brought us closer and strengthened our bond.

5. Celebrating Small Wins

Throughout my journey, I've celebrated small wins and milestones. Whether it's completing a challenging hike or mastering a new yoga pose, each achievement has been a testament to my body's resilience. These victories remind me that progress is a journey of patience and self-appreciation.

6. Exploring New Horizons

Staying active during menopause has encouraged me to explore new horizons. I've tried activities I never thought I would, like paddleboarding or salsa dancing. Embracing the unknown has added an element of excitement to my wellness journey.

7. Mind-Body Connection

Prioritizing pleasure and movement has deepened my mind-body connection. I've learned to listen to my body's cues, honor its needs, and adapt my routine accordingly. This mindful approach has allowed me to move with intention and cultivate a harmonious relationship with my body.

8. Gratitude for the Journey

Above all, my journey of staying physically active and prioritizing pleasure has been a lesson in gratitude. Gratitude for my body's capabilities, for the joy that movement brings, and for the opportunity to age with strength and vitality. It's a journey I approach with appreciation and excitement for what each day holds.

Embrace Your Unique Journey

As you navigate the path of physical activity and pleasure, remember that your journey is uniquely yours. Draw inspiration from these personal insights, and let them guide you as you create a wellness routine that resonates with your desires, needs, and aspirations. With each step you take towards prioritizing pleasure and movement, you're honoring your body's incredible capacity for growth and joy.

CHAPTER 5

Emotional Intimacy - The Heartbeat of Post-Menopausal Relationships

Exploring the Essence of Emotional Intimacy

In the landscape of post-menopausal relationships, emotional intimacy emerges as a cornerstone that holds the power to deepen connections and nurture enduring bonds. In this section, we'll delve into the significance of emotional intimacy and its transformative role in shaping relationships during and beyond menopause:

1. Beyond the Physical Realm

While physical intimacy often takes center stage, emotional intimacy reveals itself as a bridge that transcends the physical realm. It's the profound understanding, vulnerability, and shared experiences that create a tapestry of connection, fostering a deeper level of togetherness.

2. A Shelter of Trust and Safety

Emotional intimacy provides a sanctuary of trust and safety in which partners can openly express their feelings, desires, and fears. It's a space where vulnerability is met with empathy and understanding, fostering an environment where both partners can be authentic without fear of judgment.

3. Navigating Life's Changes

Menopause introduces a series of changes—physical, emotional, and psychological. Emotional intimacy becomes the compass that guides partners through these changes, allowing them to navigate the journey with empathy, patience, and a shared sense of purpose.

4. Shared Experiences and Memories

Emotional intimacy is woven through shared experiences and memories. It's the laughter that arises from recalling inside jokes, the warmth of reminiscing about milestones, and the strength that comes from facing challenges as a united front.

5. Fostering Connection Through Communication

Open and honest communication forms the backbone of emotional intimacy. Partners who engage in meaningful conversations create a fertile ground for emotional growth. By discussing hopes, dreams, and fears, they nurture a connection that goes beyond the surface.

6. Embracing Change Together

The transitions that accompany menopause invite partners to embrace change as a joint endeavor. Emotional intimacy empowers couples to support each other through these shifts, celebrating victories and extending understanding during moments of uncertainty.

7. Savoring the Present Moment

Emotional intimacy encourages partners to savor the present moment. It's the joy of sharing simple pleasures, the comfort of a lingering touch, and the reassurance that in each moment, they're cherished and valued.

8. Building Resilience

As partners navigate the challenges of menopause and life's ups and downs, emotional intimacy builds resilience. The strong foundation of connection becomes a source of strength that supports them through every twist and turn.

9. A World of Connection

Emotional intimacy weaves a tapestry of connection that grows richer with time. It's a living bond that evolves as partners deepen their understanding of each other, creating a legacy of love that enriches their lives and the lives of those around them.

Nurturing Emotional Bonds

As you journey through this chapter, remember that emotional intimacy is the heartbeat that sustains and nurtures post-menopausal relationships. By embracing its significance and fostering moments of connection, you're weaving a narrative of love, understanding, and shared growth that transcends the challenges of menopause and celebrates the beauty of partnership.

Personal Stories of Emotional Connection

Illuminating the Strength of Emotional Bonds

Allow me to share personal anecdotes that underscore the transformative power of emotional connection in post-menopausal relationships. These stories are windows into moments of vulnerability, understanding, and growth, revealing the profound impact that emotional intimacy can have:

1. The Comfort of Shared Tears

During a particularly challenging time, my partner and I found solace in each other's arms. Without words, we shared tears—tears of frustration, sadness, and mutual understanding. In that moment, the depth of our emotional connection became evident as we leaned on each other for support without judgment or explanation.

2. The Language of a Touch

One evening, my partner reached out and held my hand as we watched the sunset. No words were exchanged, yet the touch conveyed volumes—comfort, solidarity, and a shared appreciation for the beauty of the moment. It reminded me that emotional connection can transcend words and find expression in the simplest of gestures.

3. The Power of Listening

During a heart-to-heart conversation, my partner's attentive listening made me feel truly heard. As I shared my thoughts and fears, they provided a safe space for my emotions to unfold. This experience reinforced that emotional intimacy thrives when partners actively engage in listening and validation.

4. Laughter Through Tears

In the midst of a difficult conversation, a shared moment of laughter emerged. It was a reminder that emotional connection doesn't solely exist in serious discussions; it thrives in moments of shared joy and lightheartedness, even during challenging times.

5. Celebrating Small Triumphs

When I achieved a personal goal, my partner celebrated with me in a heartfelt manner. Their genuine enthusiasm mirrored the depth of our emotional bond. This experience highlighted that emotional intimacy is equally present in celebrating successes as it is in supporting during setbacks.

6. Embracing Vulnerability

Opening up about my fears and insecurities led to an unexpected outcome—my partner shared their own vulnerabilities in return. This exchange reinforced that emotional intimacy is nurtured when partners create a space where both can be authentic without fear of judgment.

7. Weathering Life's Storms

During a particularly stormy night, my partner and I watched the rain together. The metaphor of weathering the storm mirrored our journey through life's challenges. In that moment, I realized that emotional connection is about standing strong together, even when faced with adversity.

8. A Letter of Love

Receiving a heartfelt letter from my partner, filled with words of love and appreciation, touched me deeply. It was a reminder that emotional intimacy finds expression not only in spoken words but also in the written expressions of the heart.

9. Sharing Dreams and Hopes

In a moment of vulnerability, I shared my dreams and aspirations with my partner. Their unwavering support and encouragement showed me that emotional intimacy involves not only understanding but also actively nurturing each other's dreams.

Embracing Your Emotional Narrative

These personal anecdotes illuminate the tapestry of emotional connection that weaves through post-menopausal relationships. As you immerse yourself in these stories, remember that your unique experiences, moments of vulnerability, and shared joys contribute to the ongoing narrative of emotional intimacy you're building with your partner. Through these stories, you're reminded that your journey is one of connection, growth, and shared love.

Nurturing Emotional Intimacy Through Interactive Practices

Fostering emotional closeness in post-menopausal relationships involves engaging in exercises and prompts that encourage open communication, vulnerability, and shared understanding. Here, I present a selection of exercises designed to deepen your emotional connection:

1. Gratitude Exchange

Set aside time each day to share something you're grateful for with your partner. This exercise cultivates positivity and reminds you both of the small joys that enrich your lives.

2. Storytelling Nights

Designate a special evening for storytelling. Take turns sharing personal stories from your past—funny, poignant, or meaningful. This exercise creates opportunities to know each other on a deeper level.

3. The Five Love Languages

Discover each other's love languages by taking the Love Languages quiz together. Knowing how you each express and receive love can guide your efforts to foster emotional connection.

4. Shared Creative Endeavors

Engage in creative activities together, whether it's cooking a new recipe, painting, or writing a story. Collaborating on creative projects strengthens your bond through shared experiences.

5. Journaling Prompts

Use journaling prompts to explore your thoughts and feelings. Set aside time to write about your aspirations, fears, and dreams. Sharing your journal entries with each other fosters mutual understanding.

6. Role Reversal

For a day, take on each other's responsibilities or roles. This exercise helps you appreciate each other's contributions and gain insights into your partner's experiences.

7. Vision Board Creation

Create vision boards individually, focusing on your dreams and goals. Then, come together to share your boards, discussing how your aspirations align and how you can support each other.

8. The "If You Really Knew Me" Exercise

Take turns completing the sentence: "If you really knew me, you'd know..." Share personal truths that you might not have discussed before. This exercise deepens vulnerability and understanding.

9. Memory Sharing

Gather photos, mementos, and keepsakes from your journey together. Spend an evening reminiscing and sharing stories associated with these items. This exercise strengthens your emotional connection through shared memories.

10. Future Exploration

Discuss your visions for the future—both individually and as a couple. Explore where you see yourselves in five, ten, or twenty years, allowing your dreams to shape your journey together.

Nurturing Your Emotional Landscape

These exercises are pathways that lead to a richer emotional landscape in your relationship. As you engage in these practices, remember that emotional closeness is a journey of shared vulnerability, open communication, and genuine understanding. By nurturing your emotional connection, you're sowing the seeds of a relationship that flourishes with depth, empathy, and shared growth.

Overcoming Challenges - Nurturing Emotional Intimacy

Solutions for Navigating Common Challenges

Navigating the landscape of emotional intimacy in post-menopausal relationships can come with its share of challenges. Here, I offer solutions to address these common hurdles and nurture a deep and enduring emotional connection:

1. Time Constraints

Challenge: Busy schedules and responsibilities can make it difficult to prioritize emotional intimacy.

Solution: Set aside dedicated time for connection. Schedule regular date nights, even if they're at-home dinners or virtual movie nights. Creating intentional moments for each other strengthens your bond.

2. Communication Barriers

Challenge: Effective communication is essential for emotional intimacy, but miscommunication or misunderstandings can create barriers.

Solution: Practice active listening. Give your partner your full attention when they speak, and ask clarifying questions to ensure you understand their perspective. Engage in open and honest conversations about your feelings, fears, and aspirations.

3. Physical Distance

Challenge: Physical separation due to travel, work, or other commitments can strain emotional connection.

Solution: Embrace technology. Stay connected through phone calls, video chats, and text messages. Share your daily experiences, thoughts, and emotions to maintain a sense of closeness, even when apart.

4. Routine and Predictability

Challenge: Falling into a routine can lead to emotional complacency.

Solution: Inject spontaneity into your relationship. Surprise each other with thoughtful gestures, plan surprise outings, or explore new activities together. Embracing novelty keeps the spark alive.

5. Resentment or Unresolved Issues

Challenge: Lingering resentment or unresolved conflicts can hinder emotional intimacy.

Solution: Address issues as they arise. Practice active conflict resolution by listening to each other's perspectives, acknowledging feelings, and working together to find solutions. Seek professional help if necessary.

6. Prioritizing Self-Care

Challenge: Focusing on personal well-being might lead to neglecting the relationship.

Solution: Balance self-care with partner care. Prioritize individual well-being while also making time to connect. Remember that emotional intimacy thrives when both partners feel valued and supported.

7. Fear of Vulnerability

Challenge: Fear of being vulnerable can prevent open sharing of thoughts and feelings.

Solution: Lead by example. Initiate conversations where you share your own vulnerabilities and emotions. Creating a safe space encourages your partner to reciprocate, deepening emotional intimacy.

8. External Stressors

Challenge: External stressors like work, finances, or health concerns can overshadow emotional connection.

Solution: Face challenges as a team. Discuss the impact of external stressors on your relationship, share your concerns, and collaborate on strategies to manage stress together.

9. Lack of Quality Time

Challenge: Spending quality time together can be challenging with busy lives.

Solution: Make the most of everyday moments. Engage in meaningful conversations during shared activities, such as cooking, walking, or even while doing household chores together.

10. Embracing Growth Together

Challenge: People change over time, which can affect emotional intimacy.

Solution: Embrace growth as a couple. Recognize that personal growth is a natural part of life. Share your aspirations and encourage each other's development, ensuring that your emotional connection evolves with you.

Nurturing Lasting Emotional Bonds

By implementing these solutions, you're actively nurturing an emotional connection that stands strong against challenges. Remember that emotional intimacy is a dynamic journey requiring ongoing effort, understanding, and mutual support. As you face obstacles together, you're forging a relationship that grows even more resilient and meaningful with each hurdle you overcome.

CHAPTER 6

Overcoming Obstacles - Navigating Challenges in Post-Menopausal Intimacy

Identifying and Addressing Potential Obstacles

In the realm of post-menopausal intimacy, various challenges can arise that impact the emotional and physical connection between partners. In this section, we'll explore these potential obstacles and provide insights on how to navigate them, ensuring that your intimate bond remains strong and resilient:

1. Physical Changes and Discomfort

Challenge: Menopause often brings physical changes such as vaginal dryness, discomfort, or reduced libido.

Solution: Open communication is key. Discuss any physical changes openly with your partner, and consider seeking guidance from healthcare professionals. Explore various lubricants, moisturizers, and techniques that enhance comfort and pleasure.

2. Hormonal Shifts and Mood Swings

Challenge: Hormonal fluctuations during menopause can lead to mood swings and emotional changes.

Solution: Foster understanding. Both partners can educate themselves about the emotional impacts of hormonal shifts. Practice patience, empathy, and active listening to navigate mood changes with care and compassion.

3. Self-Esteem and Body Image

Challenge: Changes in body image or self-esteem can affect confidence in intimate settings.

Solution: Cultivate self-acceptance. Celebrate your body for its strength and resilience. Engage in positive self-talk and share your feelings with your partner, who can offer reassurance and support.

4. Performance Anxiety

Challenge: Concerns about performance can create anxiety and hinder intimacy.

Solution: Focus on connection. Shift the focus from performance to shared connection and emotional closeness. Prioritize open communication and mutual understanding about each other's desires and needs.

5. Lack of Communication

Challenge: Lack of communication about desires, needs, or concerns can create emotional distance.

Solution: Initiate conversations. Create an environment where both partners feel comfortable discussing intimate matters. Use "I" statements to express feelings, desires, and fears without blaming or criticizing.

6. Relationship Dynamics

Challenge: Shifts in roles and responsibilities can impact intimacy.

Solution: Redefine roles. As partners transition into different life phases, openly discuss and redefine roles to balance responsibilities and nurture the relationship. Keep the lines of communication open to ensure both partners feel valued.

7. External Stressors

Challenge: External stressors like work, family, or health concerns can impact intimacy.

Solution: Practice stress management. Develop coping strategies to manage external stressors together. Set boundaries to protect quality time for your relationship.

8. Lack of Education

Challenge: Lack of knowledge about menopause and its impact on intimacy can create uncertainty.

Solution: Educate yourselves. Seek reputable sources of information about menopause and its effects on intimacy. Attend seminars or workshops together to gain insights and strategies.

9. Routine and Predictability

Challenge: Falling into routines can lead to emotional complacency.

Solution: Embrace novelty. Engage in new activities together, try different forms of intimacy, or explore new hobbies. The element of novelty keeps the relationship fresh and exciting.

10. Seeking Professional Help

Challenge: Overcoming obstacles might require professional guidance.

Solution: Be open to seeking help. If challenges persist, consider couples therapy or seeking advice from healthcare professionals who specialize in menopause-related concerns.

Navigating Obstacles Together

By recognizing potential obstacles and proactively addressing them, you're equipping yourselves with the tools to navigate the complexities of post-menopausal intimacy. Through open communication, empathy, and a commitment to mutual growth, you're forging a path that leads to lasting intimacy, understanding, and shared fulfillment.

Real-Life Triumphs Over Challenges

Illuminating the Journeys of Resilient Couples

Let's explore the inspiring real-life stories of couples who have triumphed over challenges in post-menopausal intimacy. These stories serve as beacons of hope and examples of how dedication, communication, and mutual support can lead to a stronger and more fulfilling connection:

1. Rediscovering Passion Through Communication

John and Maria faced a decline in physical intimacy due to hormonal changes. Instead of allowing this challenge to create distance, they chose to communicate openly. They attended workshops together to learn about post-menopausal changes and explored new ways to connect emotionally and physically. By prioritizing communication, they reignited their passion and strengthened their bond.

2. Embracing Vulnerability for Deeper Connection

Sara and Alex encountered self-esteem issues that affected their intimacy. They decided to embark on a journey of self-discovery together. Through open conversations and shared activities that promoted self-acceptance, they cultivated a sense of vulnerability that deepened their emotional connection. Their journey taught them that vulnerability is the gateway to profound intimacy.

3. Healing Through Mutual Understanding

After experiencing a lack of desire, Rachel and Mark were determined to address the issue together. They sought guidance from healthcare professionals and attended counseling sessions. Through this process, they realized that emotional intimacy was as crucial as physical connection. By understanding each other's experiences and feelings, they not only revitalized their intimacy but also fostered lasting emotional closeness.

4. Rekindling Joy Amidst Change

Jenna and Chris navigated the challenges of menopause by embracing change with a sense of adventure. They embarked on a journey of trying new activities and hobbies together. By prioritizing shared experiences and novel adventures, they infused their relationship with excitement and rejuvenation, reminding each other that growth is an integral part of their journey.

5. From Struggles to Shared Triumphs

Emma and Liam faced external stressors that strained their relationship. Instead of allowing stress to drive them apart, they united against these challenges. They practiced active communication, shared their concerns openly, and developed strategies to manage stress together. Their commitment to facing adversity as a team not only strengthened their bond but also served as a testament to their enduring connection.

6. Celebrating Every Victory, Big or Small

Megan and Michael learned to celebrate every triumph, no matter how small. From conquering communication barriers to addressing physical changes, they acknowledged and celebrated each step they took together. This practice of celebrating milestones fostered a sense of accomplishment and unity, reminding them that their journey was marked by growth and shared achievements.

7. A Foundation of Friendship and Laughter

Sarah and James's success story was rooted in friendship and laughter. They faced challenges with humor and mutual support, transforming their journey into an adventure filled with shared jokes, playful moments, and genuine joy. Their bond reminded them that emotional intimacy thrives when partners are not only lovers but also best friends.

8. Mutual Empowerment Through Education

Amy and David empowered themselves with knowledge about menopause and its effects. They attended seminars, read books, and engaged in conversations with experts. By actively seeking information, they dismantled misconceptions and cultivated understanding. Their shared journey of education not only deepened their connection but also enabled them to support each other effectively.

Embracing Your Unique Journey

These real-life success stories illuminate the paths of couples who have navigated obstacles with determination, love, and shared effort. As you read about their journeys, remember that your own challenges are opportunities for growth, connection, and triumph. By drawing inspiration from these stories, you're forging a path that leads to a post-menopausal intimacy defined by resilience, understanding, and enduring love.

Empowering Solutions for Everyday Challenges

Here are practical strategies to help you navigate common concerns that may arise in post-menopausal intimacy. These strategies are designed to empower you with tools for open communication, mutual understanding, and shared growth:

1. Physical Changes and Discomfort

Concern: Addressing physical discomfort during intimacy.

Strategy: Prioritize open communication. Discuss any discomfort or changes openly with your partner. Explore different lubricants, moisturizers, or products designed to enhance comfort and pleasure. Engage in non-intimate touch and physical connection to maintain closeness.

2. Emotional Changes and Communication Barriers

Concern: Navigating mood swings and communication challenges.

Strategy: Create a safe space for open conversations. Develop a signal that indicates when one partner needs space to process emotions. Use "I" statements to express feelings and avoid blaming. Consider engaging in activities that promote relaxation and emotional well-being, such as meditation or walks.

3. Self-Esteem and Body Image

Concern: Addressing self-esteem issues related to body changes.

Strategy: Cultivate self-acceptance. Engage in positive self-talk and affirmations. Share your feelings with your partner to receive reassurance and support. Embrace activities that boost self-confidence, such as exercise or engaging in hobbies that make you feel good about yourself.

4. Performance Anxiety

Concern: Overcoming performance anxiety.

Strategy: Focus on the journey, not the outcome. Prioritize connection and shared experiences over performance. Engage in sensual activities that emphasize touch, emotional connection, and intimacy. Communicate your desires and needs openly to alleviate pressure.

5. Lack of Communication

Concern: Overcoming communication barriers.

Strategy: Schedule regular check-ins. Set aside time to discuss intimate matters, feelings, and desires. Engage in active listening and avoid interrupting each other. Use positive reinforcement to encourage open sharing and make communication a habit.

6. Routine and Predictability

Concern: Infusing novelty and excitement into the relationship.

Strategy: Plan surprise date nights or outings. Try new activities or hobbies together to introduce novelty. Experiment with new ways of intimacy that promote emotional and physical connection. Keep an open mind to trying new experiences.

7. External Stressors

Concern: Managing external stressors' impact on intimacy.

Strategy: Prioritize stress management. Engage in relaxation techniques such as deep breathing, meditation, or yoga. Create a peaceful environment for intimacy by reducing distractions. Set boundaries to protect quality time for each other.

8. Seeking Professional Help

Concern: Addressing persistent challenges that require expert guidance.

Strategy: Be open to seeking help. Consider couples therapy to facilitate productive conversations and resolutions. Consult healthcare professionals for medical concerns. Approach professional help as an opportunity for growth and mutual understanding.

9. Lack of Education

Concern: Gaining knowledge about menopause and its effects.

Strategy: Educate yourselves together. Attend seminars, workshops, or classes on menopause-related topics. Read books or articles that provide insights into the physiological and emotional aspects of menopause. Engage in conversations that foster understanding.

10. Prioritizing Emotional Connection

Concern: Nurturing emotional closeness amidst challenges.

Strategy: Create rituals of connection. Engage in activities that promote emotional intimacy, such as sharing daily highlights or engaging in intimate conversations before bed. Engage in shared activities that allow vulnerability, such as journaling or creative projects.

Thriving Through Solutions

By embracing these strategies, you're equipping yourselves with practical tools to overcome challenges and nurture your post-menopausal intimacy. Remember that every concern you face is an opportunity for growth, learning, and deepening your bond. With these strategies in hand, you're crafting a relationship defined by resilience, understanding, and a shared commitment to lasting connection.

Seeking Professional Guidance - A Balanced Perspective

Navigating the Decision to Seek Expert Help

When facing challenges in post-menopausal intimacy, the option of seeking professional guidance can offer valuable insights and support. Here, we present a balanced perspective on seeking expert help, helping you make an informed decision that aligns with your unique journey:

1. Recognizing the Value

Professional guidance can provide a fresh perspective and expert insights. Therapists, counselors, and healthcare professionals specialize in addressing challenges related to intimacy, communication, and health. Their expertise can offer solutions that you might not have considered.

2. Normalizing Challenges

Seeking help does not imply weakness or failure. Challenges are a natural part of any relationship, and professionals are equipped to guide you through them. Acknowledging the need for assistance is a sign of strength and commitment to your relationship's growth.

3. Enhancing Communication

Experts create a structured environment for communication. Couples therapy, for example, offers a safe space to address concerns and learn effective communication techniques. Professionals guide conversations and ensure both partners are heard, fostering mutual understanding.

4. Addressing Health Concerns

Healthcare professionals are equipped to address physical concerns that impact intimacy. Whether it's discussing hormonal changes, recommending treatments, or providing guidance on self-care, seeking medical help can improve both partners' well-being.

5. Timing is Key

Choose the right time to seek help. If challenges persist or escalate, professional guidance can prevent issues from worsening. However, don't wait until the situation becomes dire—early intervention can lead to quicker resolution.

6. Mutual Commitment

Couples must be on the same page about seeking help. It's crucial that both partners are open to the idea and committed to the process. Remember that seeking professional guidance is a joint decision that requires mutual agreement.

7. Confidentiality and Safety

Professional settings provide confidentiality, ensuring that your concerns remain private. This safe space encourages open sharing without fear of judgment or repercussions. It's an opportunity to discuss sensitive matters openly.

8. Continuous Learning

Sessions with experts offer valuable skills that extend beyond addressing immediate concerns. You'll acquire tools for effective communication, conflict resolution, and emotional connection that will benefit your relationship long-term.

9. Building Strong Foundations

Seeking help reinforces your commitment to the relationship. It's an investment in creating a strong foundation for the future. By actively working on challenges, you're building a relationship that thrives through mutual growth and understanding.

10. The Decision is Yours

Ultimately, the decision to seek professional guidance is a personal one. Reflect on your needs, concerns, and goals. If you both feel that seeking help aligns with your journey, remember that it's a positive step toward nurturing your intimacy and creating a more fulfilling relationship.

Making Informed Choices

When considering seeking professional guidance, weigh the benefits, timing, and mutual commitment carefully. Whether you decide to engage in therapy, counseling, or medical consultation, remember that your goal is to create a relationship defined by connection, understanding, and shared growth. Seeking help is a proactive choice that demonstrates your dedication to building a resilient and thriving post-menopausal intimacy.

CHAPTER 7

Celebrating Connection - Reflections on the Writing Journey

Embracing the Journey and Gaining Insights

In this section, we embark on a reflective journey through the process of writing this book and the insights gained along the way. The path to creating "The Post-Menopause Sex Guide: How to Stay Intimate and Satisfied" has been a transformative one, filled with discoveries, growth, and a deeper understanding of the topics explored:

From the very first moment of conceptualizing this book, the journey has been one of both excitement and challenges. The title itself embodies the essence of the content within—addressing the intricacies of post-menopausal intimacy and guiding readers toward lasting connection and satisfaction.

1. A Vision Takes Shape

As I envisioned crafting a guide that would offer practical solutions and emotional support, the blueprint for each chapter began to take form. The goal was not only to provide information but to create a genuine connection with readers, resonating with their experiences and concerns.

2. Research and Realization

Researching the topics of menopause, intimacy, and relationships brought a wealth of knowledge and insights. The journey revealed the diverse experiences individuals face during this phase of life, and it became clear that a personalized approach was essential to addressing their unique needs.

3. Balancing Information and Emotion

Striking a balance between informative discourse and emotional connection became a central theme. Each chapter sought to provide accurate information while infusing personal anecdotes, real-life stories, and relatable examples that readers could connect with on a deeply human level.

4. Growth Through Empathy

The writing journey fostered empathy, as I delved into the challenges individuals and couples encounter during post-menopausal years. Personal stories shared by readers and my own experiences lent a deeper understanding of the emotional landscape, reinforcing the importance of emotional intimacy.

5. Strengthening the Author-Reader Bond

The process of crafting introductions, main ideas, and subsections was not merely an exercise in organization; it was a way to build a connection with readers. Each chapter aimed to engage, enlighten, and empower, drawing readers into a dialogue that transcends the pages.

6. The Joy of Solutions

Sharing practical strategies, exercises, and real-life success stories underscored the solutions-focused approach. Every piece of advice was crafted to empower readers, reminding them that they have the agency to nurture their intimacy and relationship.

7. Gratitude and Fulfillment

As the book neared completion, gratitude filled my heart—for the opportunity to contribute to readers' lives, for the lessons learned, and for the connections formed through shared stories and experiences. The journey of writing this guide has been a celebration of connection in itself.

Section 2: Embracing Insights and Continuing the Journey

Reflecting on the journey of writing "The Post-Menopause Sex Guide," we have gained not only insights into the topics explored but also a deeper appreciation for the power of connection, vulnerability, and growth. As readers embark on their own journeys with this guide, may they find inspiration in the shared path toward intimacy, satisfaction, and the celebration of meaningful connections.

A Personal Journey of Growth and

Transformation

A Story of Personal Evolution

As the journey of writing "The Post-Menopause Sex Guide" unfolded, it paralleled a transformative chapter in my own life. Through the process of researching, crafting, and sharing insights, I too experienced growth and transformation, learning lessons that have enriched my understanding of intimacy, connection, and personal development:

1. Embracing Vulnerability

Writing a guide that delves into the nuances of intimacy required vulnerability. Just as the guide encourages readers to open up and connect, I found myself embracing vulnerability in my writing process. This shift allowed me to share personal anecdotes, insights, and experiences that fostered a genuine connection with readers.

2. Overcoming Doubts

Challenges arose, much like the obstacles discussed in the book. Doubts about my ability to provide valuable insights and engage readers sometimes crept in. Yet, just as I advised readers to overcome their doubts, I employed the same strategies—self-compassion, seeking guidance, and reminding myself of my unique perspective.

3. Rediscovering Passion

Through the chapters on rediscovering desire, I too underwent a process of reigniting passion. Not just in the realm of intimacy, but in the journey of creation. I felt a renewed sense of purpose as I explored the topics, uncovering the joy of sharing meaningful content with others.

4. Cultivating Connection

The chapters on communication resonated deeply, inspiring me to apply the lessons to my own relationships. I engaged in open conversations with loved ones, fostered deeper connections, and learned that the skills discussed in the book can be transformative in various aspects of life.

5. Honoring Personal Growth

The journey of writing this guide reinforced the importance of continuous personal growth. Just as I urged readers to embrace change and self-discovery, I embraced growth in my own life. This journey enriched my perspective and deepened my commitment to offering meaningful content.

6. Celebrating Milestones

Each chapter's completion became a milestone worth celebrating—a testament to dedication, perseverance, and a commitment to helping others. These victories reminded me of the power of progress and the importance of celebrating even the smallest steps forward.

7. An Ongoing Journey

The journey of writing this guide is far from over. Just as the book is a guide for readers, the process itself has guided my own growth. As I reflect on my personal journey, I'm reminded that transformation is a continuous process, and every step taken brings us closer to a more fulfilled and connected life.

Nurturing Growth in Unity

The personal transformation that unfolded during the creation of this guide is a testament to the power of growth, connection, and shared insights. As you engage with the content and embark on your own journey of growth and transformation, may the lessons shared here inspire you to embrace vulnerability, overcome challenges, and celebrate the joy of connection.

Key Takeaways - A Journey of Insights

Unveiling Essential Lessons

In this section, we distill the essential takeaways from each chapter of "The Post-Menopause Sex Guide," offering a concise summary of the key insights that will guide you on your path to intimacy, connection, and personal growth:

Chapter 1: Embracing Change

Takeaway: Menopause brings physical and emotional changes. Embrace them as opportunities for growth and connection. Address common misconceptions and societal perceptions that can hinder intimacy.

Chapter 2: Navigating Communication

Takeaway: Open communication is the cornerstone of intimacy. Prioritize honest conversations, share feelings, and use active listening to foster understanding.

Chapter 3: Rediscovering Desire

Takeaway: Desire evolves during menopause. Utilize relatable metaphors to understand this evolution. Rediscover desire through personal insights, shared experiences, and purposeful activities.

Chapter 4: Physical Well-being and Pleasure

Takeaway: Physical well-being enhances intimacy. Incorporate health and fitness insights to maintain vitality. Engage in exercises that promote pleasure and comfort.

Chapter 5: Emotional Intimacy

Takeaway: Emotional intimacy is essential. Share personal anecdotes that highlight the power of emotional connection. Foster closeness through exercises and address common challenges.

Chapter 6: Overcoming Obstacles

Takeaway: Challenges are normal. Address potential obstacles by embracing open communication, prioritizing self-care, and seeking professional guidance when needed.

Chapter 7: Celebrating Connection

Takeaway: Reflect on your journey. Understand the insights gained through writing and personal growth. Embrace vulnerability, overcome doubts, and celebrate milestones.

Navigating Your Personal Path

As you carry these key takeaways with you, remember that each chapter is a stepping stone on your journey. From embracing change and rediscovering desire to nurturing emotional intimacy and overcoming challenges, every insight is a tool that empowers you to create a fulfilling and lasting post-menopausal connection.

Your Journey, Your Triumphs

In this section, we invite you to embrace the progress you've made and actively foster connection within your relationships. As you navigate the path outlined in "The Post-Menopause Sex Guide," remember that every step forward is a triumph worth celebrating:

1. Celebrate Small Wins

Acknowledge and celebrate the small victories along your journey. Whether it's an open conversation, a shared experience, or a moment of vulnerability, each step contributes to your growth and connection.

2. Embrace Self-Compassion

Be kind to yourself as you navigate challenges and changes. Just as you would offer support and encouragement to a friend, extend the same compassion to yourself. Embrace your journey as a testament to your strength and resilience.

3. Share Your Progress

Share your progress with your partner or loved ones. Openly communicate about your experiences, insights, and lessons learned. Sharing creates a space for mutual understanding and fosters a deeper connection.

4. Create Rituals of Connection

Incorporate rituals that nurture connection into your routine. Whether it's a weekly date night, a daily check-in, or a shared activity, these rituals strengthen the bond between you and your partner.

5. Prioritize Intimacy

Prioritize intimate moments that align with your desires and comfort level. Whether it's physical intimacy, emotional closeness, or simply spending quality time together, these moments contribute to a deeper connection.

6. Seek Adventure Together

Embark on new adventures as a couple. Whether it's trying a new activity, exploring a new place, or engaging in a shared hobby, novelty keeps the relationship exciting and fosters growth.

7. Reflect on Progress

Periodically reflect on how far you've come. Review the insights you've gained, the challenges you've overcome, and the connections you've deepened. Recognize your growth as a continuous journey.

8. Cultivate Gratitude

Practice gratitude for the journey you're on and the connections you're nurturing. Express appreciation for your partner's support, the lessons you've learned, and the shared moments that enrich your relationship.

9. Celebrate Milestones

Mark significant milestones with joy and celebration. Whether it's an anniversary, a shared achievement, or simply a moment of emotional connection, use these milestones as opportunities to commemorate your journey.

10. Embrace the Journey

Remember that your journey is uniquely yours. Embrace the highs and the challenges, for each experience contributes to your growth and connection. Your commitment to fostering intimacy and connection is a testament to the love you share.

Thriving in Connection

As you journey forward, carry these encouragements with you. Celebrate the progress you make, nurture connection, and continue to explore the depths of intimacy. With each step, you're shaping a relationship that thrives in the embrace of growth, understanding, and shared connection.

CONCLUSION

Nurturing Your Path of Intimacy

Your Journey, Your Connection

As we reach the end of "The Post-Menopause Sex Guide: How to Stay Intimate and Satisfied," I want to extend my heartfelt encouragement and support to each and every reader who has embarked on this journey. Your commitment to nurturing post-menopausal intimacy is a testament to your strength, resilience, and unwavering love.

Throughout these chapters, we've explored the intricacies of post-menopausal intimacy, delved into the nuances of communication, rediscovered desire, prioritized well-being, and nurtured emotional connection. Every word written was crafted with the hope of guiding you toward a deeper understanding of yourself, your partner, and the beautiful connection you share.

As you navigate the challenges and joys of this phase of life, remember that you possess the ability to overcome obstacles, embrace change, and foster meaningful connections. The insights shared within these pages are not just words—they are tools that empower you to create a post-menopausal journey defined by growth, closeness, and fulfillment.

I want to express my deepest gratitude for allowing me to be a part of your journey. The opportunity to provide guidance and support has been an honor, and I am humbled by the stories you've shared, the progress you've made, and the connections you've deepened. Your willingness to engage with this guide demonstrates your commitment to growth and your desire to nurture a lasting and thriving connection.

As you move forward, remember that post-menopausal intimacy is a continuous journey, one filled with moments of growth, shared laughter, and cherished connection. Embrace vulnerability, celebrate your progress, and continue to explore the depths of love that flourish when partners support, learn from, and cherish each other.

May your path be illuminated by the insights gained, and may your connection thrive in the embrace of understanding and compassion. Your journey is uniquely yours, and I have full confidence that you will navigate it with grace and determination.

With warmth, support, and gratitude,

[Amara Adams]

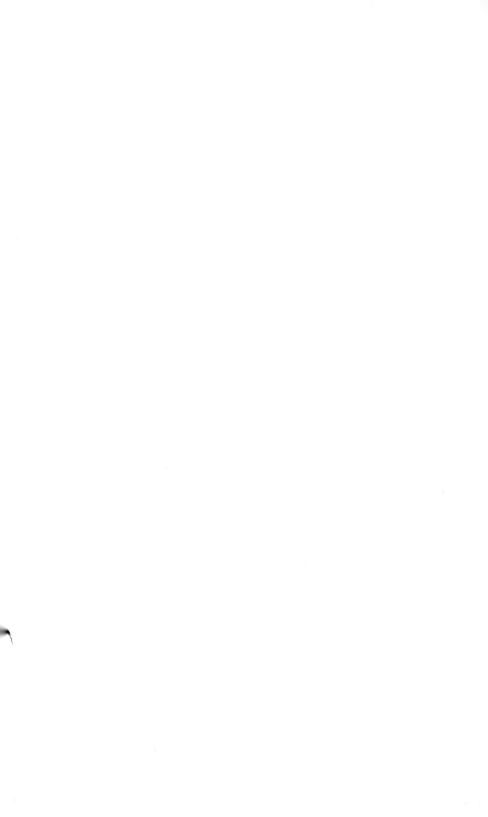

Made in United States
Troutdale, OR
12/29/2023

16528965R00046